RADIANT BALANCE:
Nurturing Your Oily Skin Naturally

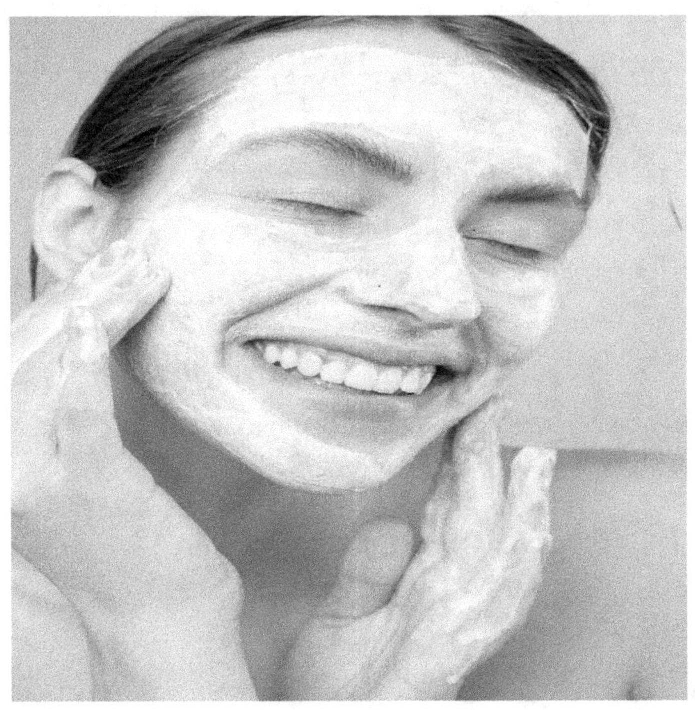

A Comprehensive Guide To Oily Skin Care Using Natural Ingredients

TABLE OF CONTENT

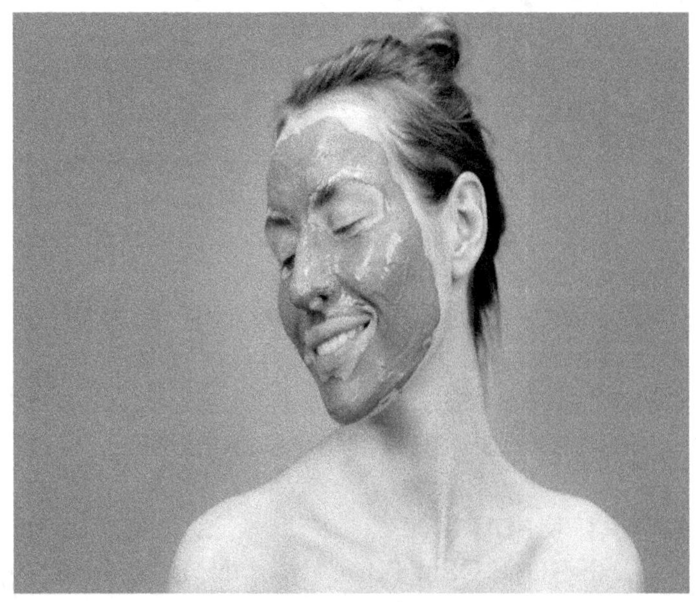

INTRODUCTION

In the quest for radiant and healthy skin, individuals with oily skin often find themselves struggling with excess shine, enlarged pores and occasional breakouts.
Oily skin can be a challenge to manage, but with the right skincare routine, you can achieve a healthy, balanced complexion skin.

 The good news is that nature provides an arsenal of ingredients that can help manage oily skin without resorting to harsh chemicals that may be damaging to the skin.

Natural skincare is becoming increasingly popular because it focuses on using ingredients derived from nature, free from harsh chemicals, to promote skin health.
When it comes to oily skin, the goal is to control excess oil production, prevent breakouts, and maintain a clear and radiant complexion.

This book provides a comprehensive guide to natural skincare for oily skin, covering everything from understanding your skin type to a guide through the world of natural skincare for oily skin creating your own skincare products and shedding light on ingredients that can take care of your common skin concerns and those that may cause more harm than good.

Here's an introduction to natural skincare for oily skin:

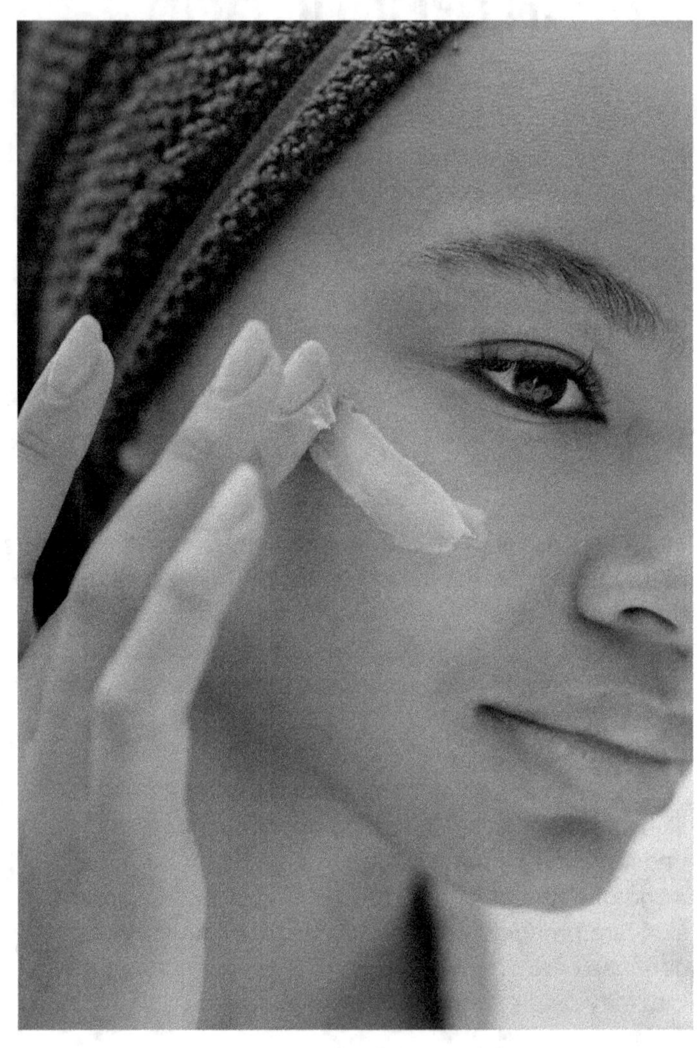

CHAPTER ONE

WHAT'S MY SKIN TYPE?

Identifying your skin type is essential for selecting the right skincare products and routines.
There are four primary skin types: normal, oily, dry, and combination.

Here's how to identify your skin type:
The Bare-Faced Test:
Start with a clean face. Use a mild, sulfate-free cleanser to remove any makeup or products from your skin.
Pat your face dry gently with a clean towel.
Leave your skin bare (without applying any skincare products) for a few hours or even a full day.

Observation:
After some time has passed, observe how your skin feels and looks.
Normal Skin:
If your skin feels comfortable, not too dry or too oily, and looks clear without noticeable dry patches or excessive shine, you likely have normal skin.
Oily Skin:
If your skin appears shiny, especially in the T-zone (forehead, nose, and chin), and you may notice enlarged pores or occasional acne breakouts, you probably have oily skin.
Dry Skin:
If your skin feels tight, rough, or flaky, and you experience dry patches or redness, you likely have dry skin.

Combination Skin:
If you notice that some areas of your face are oily (usually the T-zone) while others are dry (typically the cheeks), you may have combination skin.
Sensitive Skin:
If your skin frequently experiences redness, irritation, burning, or itching, you have sensitive skin. This can occur in combination with any of the other skin types.
Mature Skin:
As you age, your skin may change. Mature skin often becomes drier and may show fine lines and wrinkles.
Remember that your skin type can vary in different seasons and under the influence of factors like climate, diet, and lifestyle. It's also essential to consider any specific skin concerns or conditions, like acne, rosacea, or eczema, when selecting skincare products.
Once you've determined your skin type, you can tailor your skincare routine to address its specific needs. For example, oily skin may benefit from oil-free and mattifying products, while dry skin requires hydration and moisturization. If you have concerns about your skin type or specific skincare issues, it's advisable to consult a dermatologist or skincare professional for personalized recommendations.

UNDERSTANDING OILY SKIN

Oily skin is a prevalent skin type defined by an excess of sebum, the skin's natural oil.
Sebum is produced by sebaceous glands in the skin and plays a crucial role in keeping the skin hydrated and protected. However, when sebum production becomes excessive, it can lead to oily skin, which can have both positive and negative effects.

Key points to understand about oily skin:

Causes: Oily skin can be caused by various factors, including genetics, hormonal fluctuations (common during puberty, menstruation, and pregnancy), high humidity, and the use of certain skincare products.

Features: Shiny skin is a characteristic of oily skin, especially in the T-zone (forehead, nose, and chin). It could be more prone to acne and blackheads and have enlarged pores. To the touch, oily skin may feel greasy.

Advantages: Oily skin tends to age more slowly than dry skin because the natural oils help keep the skin moisturized and prevent the early formation of fine lines and wrinkles.

Challenges: Oily skin is more prone to acne and breakouts. Excess sebum can clog pores, leading to whiteheads, blackheads, and pimples. Oily skin can also make makeup less stable and lead to a shiny appearance throughout the day.

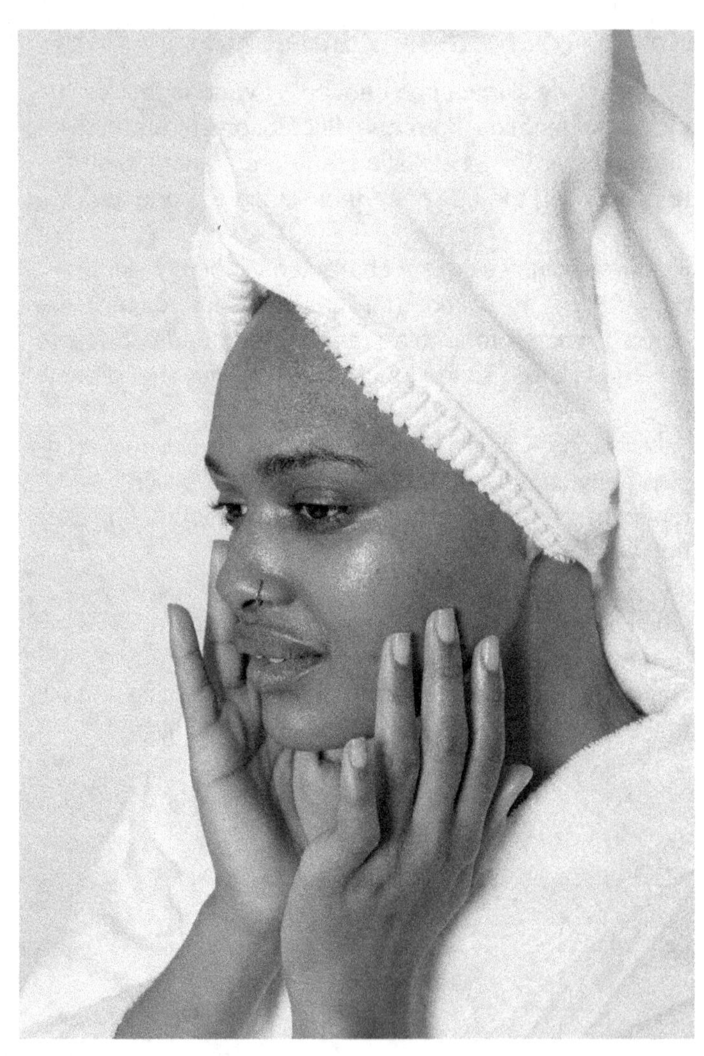

CHAPTER TWO

MANAGING OILY SKIN

To manage oily skin, it's essential to follow a proper skincare routine. This should include:
Cleansing: Use a gentle, foaming cleanser to remove excess oil and impurities without over-drying.

Toning: Use a toner with ingredients like salicylic acid or witch hazel to help balance oil production and minimize pore size.

Moisturizing: Even oily skin needs hydration. Use a lightweight, oil-free, or non-comedogenic moisturizer to prevent the skin from overcompensating with more oil production.

Sunscreen: Always wear a broad-spectrum sunscreen to protect the skin from UV damage. Look for a non-comedogenic or oil-free option.

Exfoliation: Regular exfoliation with products containing salicylic acid or glycolic acid can help remove dead skin cells and prevent clogged pores.

Diet and Lifestyle: Diet and lifestyle factors can also influence oily skin. A balanced diet, staying hydrated, and managing stress can help maintain skin health.

Professional Help: If you're struggling with severe acne or excessive oil production, it's a good idea to consult a dermatologist. They can advise you on prescription treatments or procedures to help you manage your skin.

Remember that everyone's skin is different, and what works for one person may not work for another.

Finding the right skincare routine for oily skin may involve some trial and error, but with patience and the right products, you can manage excess oil and maintain healthy, clear and radiant skin.

DAILY SKINCARE ROUTINE

A daily skincare routine for oily skin should focus on managing excess oil production, preventing breakouts, and maintaining clear, healthy skin. Here's a step-by-step guide to a basic daily skincare routine for oily skin:

Morning Routine:

Cleanser: Start your morning routine with a gentle, foaming cleanser formulated for oily skin. This will help remove any excess oil and impurities without stripping your skin of essential moisture. Rinse with lukewarm water.

Toner: Use a gentle, alcohol-free toner to balance your skin's pH levels. Toners can help reduce oiliness and prepare your skin for the next steps.

Serum (Optional): You can use a lightweight, oil-free serum with ingredients like niacinamide or salicylic acid to target specific skin concerns like acne or enlarged pores. Be sure to apply it evenly.

Moisturizer: Even if you have oily skin, it's essential to use a non-comedogenic, oil-free moisturizer. This helps

maintain skin hydration without clogging pores.
Gel-based moisturizers are a good option.

Sunscreen: Regardless of the weather, apply a
broad-spectrum, SPF 30 or higher sunscreen every
morning. Look for an oil-free sunscreen that is labeled
"non-comedogenic."

Evening Routine:

Cleanser: Use the same gentle cleanser you used in the
morning to remove makeup, dirt, and excess oil from
your skin.

Toner: To balance the pH of your skin, repeat the toner
step.

Exfoliation (2-3 times a week): Exfoliate with a chemical
exfoliant that contains salicylic acid (BHA) or glycolic
acid (AHA). This helps to unclog pores and remove dead
skin cells. Be careful not to over-exfoliate, as it can lead
to increased oil production.

Serum (Optional): If you're using a serum with specific
skin concerns, apply it after exfoliation.

Spot Treatment: Use salicylic acid or benzoyl peroxide
as a spot treatment for active breakouts.
Moisturizer: Apply the same non-comedogenic
moisturizer you used in the morning.

Additional Tips:
Use oil-free and non-comedogenic makeup products if
you wear makeup.

Blotting papers can help control excess oil during the day without removing makeup.
Keep your hands off your face to avoid transferring dirt and oil to your skin.
Stay hydrated and maintain a balanced diet to help manage oil production.
Change your pillowcases regularly to prevent the buildup of oil and bacteria.
Remember that consistency is key in skincare, and it may take time to see improvements. If you experience severe or persistent skin issues, consult a dermatologist for personalized advice and treatment options.

WEEKLY SKINCARE REGIMEN

In addition to your daily skincare routine for oily skin, incorporating a weekly skincare routine can help address specific concerns and give your skin a deeper cleanse. Here's a suggested weekly skincare routine for oily skin:
 Weekly Deep Cleansing:

Exfoliation (1-2 times a week): Use a gentle physical exfoliator (scrub) or a chemical exfoliant with alpha hydroxy acids (AHAs) like glycolic acid or beta hydroxy acids (BHAs) like salicylic acid. This aids in the removal of dead skin cells and the unclogging of pores. Avoid over-exfoliation, which can irritate the skin and increase oil production.

Clay Mask (1-2 times a week): Apply a clay mask to absorb excess oil and impurities. Clay masks can help tighten pores and reduce shine. Rinse it off thoroughly once it dries.

Pore Care:
Pore Strips (Optional): If you have visible blackheads on your nose or other areas, you can use pore strips to help remove them. Use them sparingly and follow the instructions.

Hydration and Repair:
Sheet Mask (1-2 times a week): Choose a hydrating sheet mask with ingredients like hyaluronic acid or soothing ingredients like aloe vera. This can aid in achieving a moisture balance for your skin.

Sun Protection:
Sunscreen Reapplication: If you spend an extended time outdoors, be sure to reapply sunscreen every two hours, especially during peak sun exposure hours.

Additional Tips:
Be gentle with your skin, even when using exfoliants and masks. Overzealous scrubbing can irritate the skin and exacerbate oiliness.
Before applying masks or exfoliants, do a patch test to ensure your skin can tolerate them.
Remember to adjust your weekly routine based on your skin's specific needs and sensitivities. If your skin becomes dry or irritated, reduce the frequency of certain treatments.
A well-balanced weekly skincare routine for oily skin helps maintain clear, healthy skin by addressing excess oil and preventing breakouts. Keep in mind that skincare products should be chosen based on your individual skin concerns and sensitivities. If you're uncertain about which products are suitable for your skin, consult a dermatologist for personalized advice.

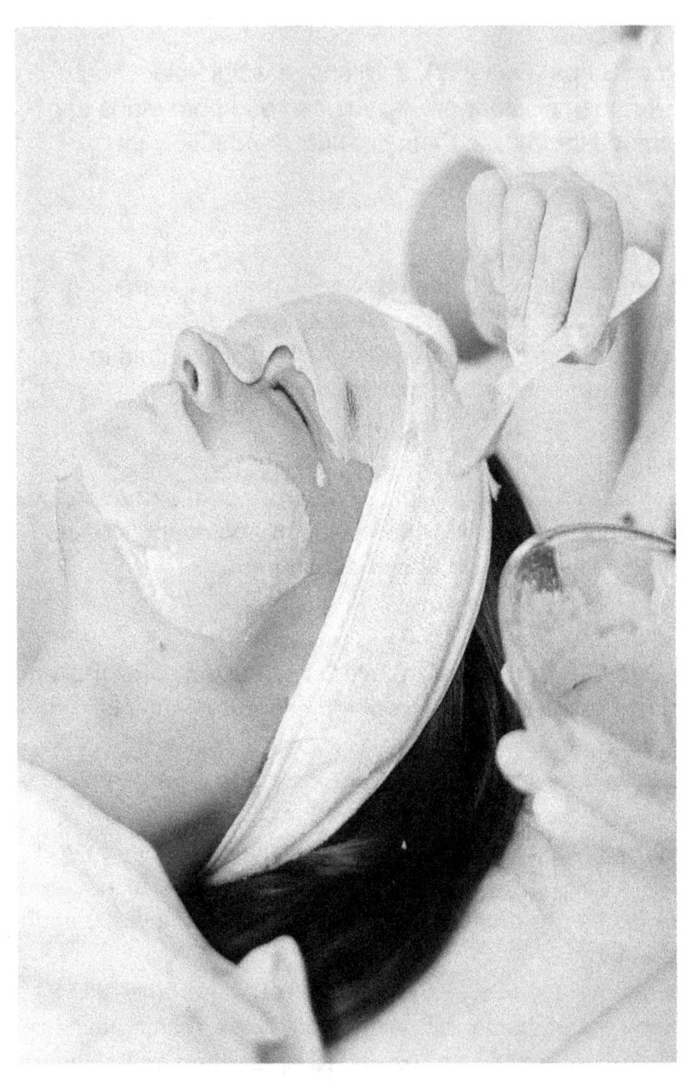

CHAPTER THREE

THE BASICS OF NATURAL SKINCARE

Natural skincare is a holistic approach to taking care of your skin using products and practices that are derived from or inspired by nature. It emphasizes using ingredients that are minimally processed and avoiding harsh chemicals and synthetic compounds. Here are the basics of natural skincare:

Cleansing: Start with a gentle natural cleanser to remove dirt, makeup, and impurities from your skin. Options include oils like coconut or jojoba oil, honey, or aloe vera.

Exfoliation: Use natural exfoliants like sugar, salt, oatmeal, or finely ground seeds to remove dead skin cells. Exfoliation helps to unclog pores and promote skin renewal.

Toning: Natural toners like rose water, witch hazel, or green tea can help balance your skin's pH levels and tighten pores.

Moisturizing: To moisturize your skin, use natural oils like jojoba, coconut, or argan. Aloe vera gel and shea butter are two more fantastic natural moisturizers.

Sun Protection: Use natural sunscreen with ingredients like zinc oxide or titanium dioxide to protect your skin from harmful UV rays.

Masks: You can create DIY masks using ingredients like honey, yogurt, clay, or oatmeal to address specific skin concerns. Masks can hydrate, detoxify, or soothe your skin.

Serums: Natural serums with ingredients like vitamin C (from citrus fruits), hyaluronic acid (found in the body), or rosehip oil can target specific skin issues and provide additional nourishment.

Diet and Hydration: What you eat and drink plays a significant role in your skin's health. Consume a balanced diet rich in fruits, vegetables, and water to support your skin from the inside.

Hygiene: Ensure that your skincare tools and containers are clean to prevent the growth of harmful bacteria.

Lifestyle: Stress management, adequate sleep, and regular exercise all contribute to the health of your skin. Skin health is often reflective of your overall well-being.

Patch Test: When trying new natural skincare products or ingredients, perform a patch test to check for any allergic reactions or sensitivities.

Consult a Dermatologist: If you have specific skin concerns or recurring problems, make an appointment with a dermatologist. They can provide guidance and recommend natural or prescription solutions.

Remember that natural skincare is about using ingredients that are kind to your skin and avoiding harsh chemicals and synthetic additives. What works best for your skin may vary, so it's important to understand your skin type and its unique needs. Additionally, be patient, as natural skincare often takes time to show noticeable results.

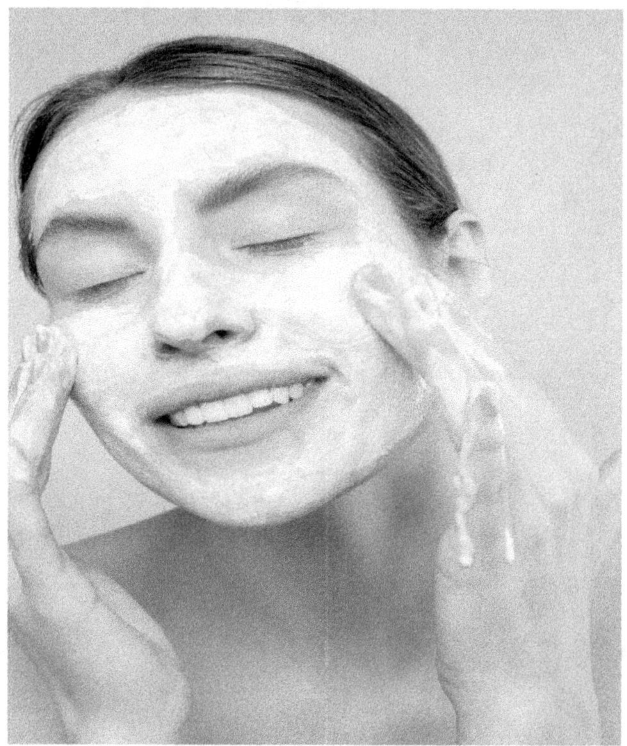

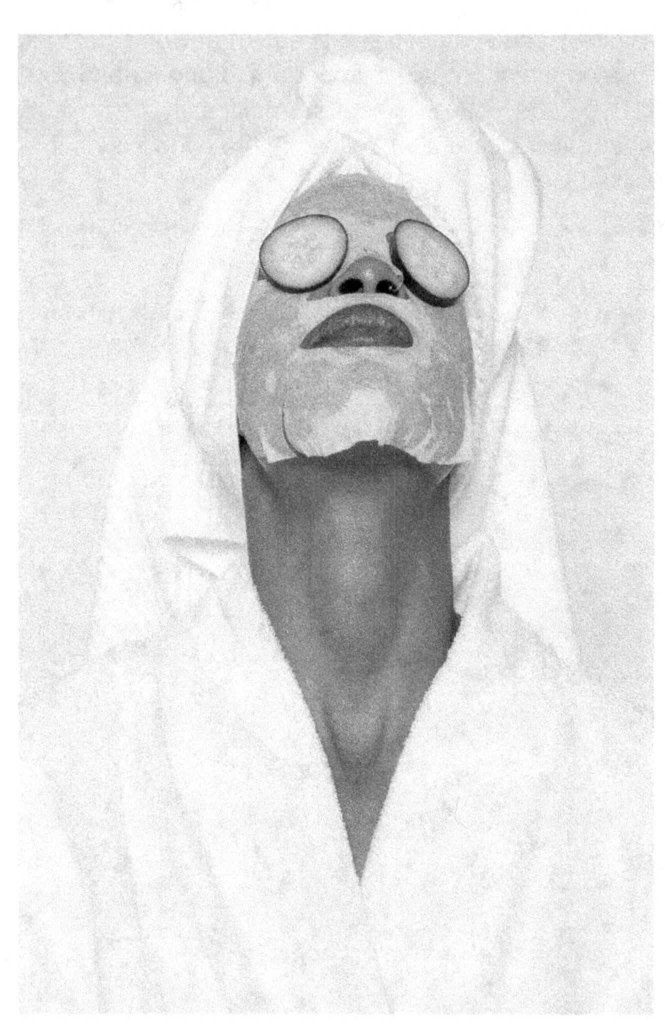

CHAPTER FOUR

THE ROLE OF pH BALANCE IN SKINCARE

The role of pH balance in skincare is crucial for maintaining healthy and radiant skin. pH stands for "potential of hydrogen" and is a measurement of the acidity or alkalinity of a substance on a scale from 0 to 14, with 7 being neutral. Skin has a natural pH level that falls in the range of 4.5 to 5.5, which is slightly acidic. Here's why pH balance is important in skincare:

Skin Barrier Function: The skin's pH level plays a vital role in maintaining its barrier function. The acid mantle, a thin, protective film on the skin's surface, helps prevent the intrusion of harmful microorganisms, allergens, and pollutants. When the pH is within the optimal range, the acid mantle functions effectively, protecting the skin from damage.

Microbiome Balance: The skin's pH level also influences the balance of the skin microbiome. Healthy skin has a diverse ecosystem of beneficial bacteria that help protect against harmful pathogens. Maintaining the right pH helps support the growth of these beneficial bacteria.

Skin Hydration: The skin's pH affects its ability to retain moisture. An acidic pH helps the skin retain water and stay adequately hydrated. Deviations from the optimal pH range can lead to skin dryness or excessive oiliness.

Skin Conditions: Imbalances in pH can exacerbate certain skin conditions. For example, excessively alkaline products can disrupt the skin's natural pH, leading to conditions like eczema or acne. On the other hand, overly acidic products can cause irritation and sensitivity.

Product Efficacy: The pH of skincare products can impact their efficacy. Some active ingredients work optimally within specific pH ranges. Using products with a pH that is too high or too low for a particular ingredient can reduce its effectiveness.

To maintain proper pH balance in your skincare routine:

Choose pH-Balanced Products: Look for cleansers, toners, and moisturizers that are formulated to be pH-balanced for the skin. These products help maintain the skin's natural pH.

Avoid Harsh Cleansers: Harsh cleansers with high pH levels can strip the skin of its natural oils and disrupt the acid mantle. Opt for gentle, pH-balanced cleansers.

Be Mindful of Exfoliants: Chemical exfoliants (e.g., AHAs and BHAs) typically have specific pH requirements for optimal results. Follow product instructions to avoid over exfoliating or ineffective exfoliation.
Patch Test: If introducing new skincare products, consider patch testing to ensure that they do not cause irritation or disrupt your skin's pH.

Personalize Your Routine: Keep in mind that everyone's skin is unique, and what works for one person may not

work for another. Adjust your skincare routine to suit
your skin's specific needs and sensitivities.

Maintaining the pH balance of your skin is an important
aspect of a healthy skincare routine. It can help keep
your skin looking and feeling its best while reducing the
risk of irritation and skin issues.

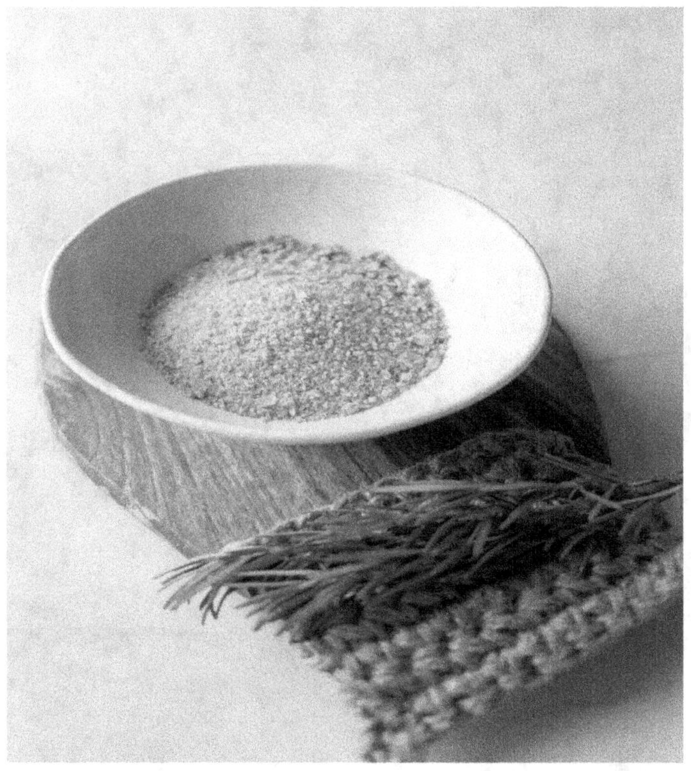

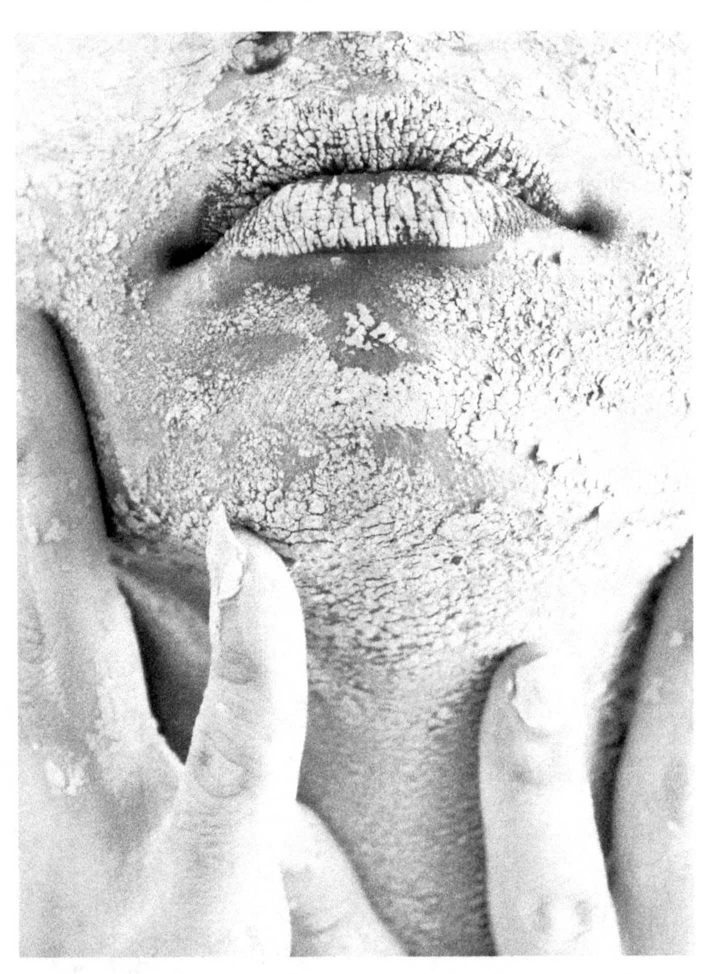

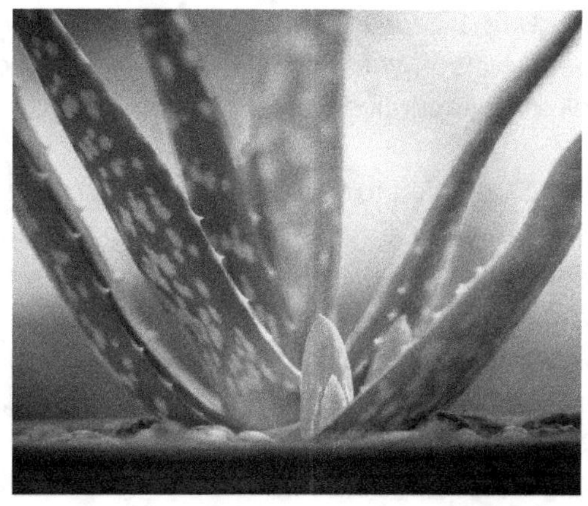

CHAPTER FIVE

NATURAL INGREDIENTS FOR OILY SKIN

Oily skin can benefit from natural ingredients that help regulate oil production, minimize pores, and keep the skin balanced and healthy. Here are some natural ingredients that are known to be effective for oily skin:

➤ *Witch Hazel:* Witch hazel is one of the natural ingredients often used in skincare routines, especially for people with oily skin. Its astringent properties can help tighten and tone the skin.
Let's outline some of the few ways you can incorporate witch hazel into your oily skincare routine:

Cleansing: Use a gentle facial cleanser infused with Witch hazel to clean your face. This will help remove dirt, excess oil, and impurities from your skin.

Toning: When applied to the face, witch hazel has a toning effect on the skin and can also help tighten pores and reduce excess oil production due to its astringent properties. Apply Witch hazel to a cotton pad (Dilute with water for sensitive skin) and gently swipe it across your face. However, be careful not to overuse witch hazel to avoid excessive drying of the skin.

Blemish and Acne treatment : Witch hazel can also be applied as a spot treatment for Blemishes and Acne. Dab a small amount on the affected areas to help reduce inflammation and redness.

NOTE: In as much as witch hazel is beneficial to those with oily skin, it may not be suitable for everyone. Some individuals may find it too harsh, drying, or even allergenic. Therefore, it is advised that you perform a patch test on a small area of your skin before using it on your entire face. More importantly, if you have any specific concern, don't hesitate to consult with a dermatologist.

➤ *Tea Tree Oil:* Tea tree oil has natural antimicrobial properties that can help with acne and excess oil. Before applying it to the skin, make sure to dilute it.
Due to its natural antimicrobial properties which has the ability to help manage excess oil production and fight acne-causing bacteria, Tea tree oil can be a useful addition to an oily skincare routine. However, Tea tree oil is highly concentrated so it should be properly diluted before use to avoid skin irritation.

Dilution: To formulate a safe and effective solution, mix a few drops (typically 1-2 drops) of tea tree oil with a carrier oil like coconut oil, grapeseed oil or jojoba oil. Dilution ratio of 1-2% tea tree oil to carrier oil.

Tips for incorporating tea tree oil into your oily skincare routine:

Cleanser: Add a few drops of diluted tea tree oil to your facial cleanser. This can help fight acne-causing bacteria and control excess oil on the skin. Be not to overuse it to avoid excessive skin dryness.

Spot Treatment: Gently apply a little amount of diluted Tea tree oil with your fingertip or using a cotton swab directly to the pimple.

Face Masks: Few drops of diluted tea tree oil added to your face masks can help control oil and treat acne.

Moisturizer: You can mix a few drops of diluted tea tree oil in your oil-free moisturizer. This can provide the benefits of tea tree oil without over-drying your skin.

Patience: When incorporating tea tree oil into your skincare routine, it's important to be patient and consistent. Results may not be immediate, and it can take time to see improvements in acne and oil control.

Patch Test: Before applying tea tree oil to your face, perform a patch test on a small area of skin to ensure you don't experience any adverse reactions or irritation.

Sun Protection: Tea tree oil may increase your skin's sensitivity to the sun. Always use sunscreen when going outside, especially if you're using tea tree oil in your routine.

Use Moderately: When it comes to tea tree oil, less really is more. Excessive use can result in skin irritation or dryness. Do not use more than the suggested dilution ratios.

See a Dermatologist: It's a good idea to see a dermatologist if you have severe or enduring acne or other skin conditions. They can offer you individualized guidance and options for treatment based on your unique requirements.

➢ **Aloe Vera**: Aloe vera is a versatile and natural ingredient that can provide a wide range of benefits for your skin. With its soothing and hydrating effect, it can help reduce redness and inflammation while providing light moisture to the skin.

Below are various ways you can use Aloe gel:

Cleanser: Aloe vera gel can be used as a gentle cleanser. Apply a little quantity of the gel to your face, massage it in, leave it on for a few minutes then rinse off with clean water.

Moisturizer: Apply a thin layer of aloe vera gel to your face as a lightweight moisturizer. It's particularly beneficial for oily or acne-prone skin.

Face Mask: Mix aloe vera gel with ingredients like honey or yogurt to formulate a hydrating face mask. Leave it on for 10 to 15 minutes, rinse it off with water.

For oily and Acne-prone skin: Mix aloe vera gel with a few drops of tea tree oil, apply a thin layer on the face or areas with acne. Aloe vera contains antibacterial and anti-inflammatory properties that are very beneficial to oily and acne-prone skin.

Aloe Vera Toner: Mix the aloe vera gel with rosewater to formulate a natural toner. Store it in a spray bottle and spray it on your face after cleansing. This helps to balance your skin's pH and also provides hydration.

Aloe Vera Scrub: Formulate a mild exfoliating scrub with Aloe vera gel by mixing gel with a little quantity of sugar or smoothly ground oatmeal. Massage the mixture gently on your face, then rinse off with clean water.

NOTE: You can use pure aloe vera gel directly from the plant or buy a high-quality, pure aloe vera gel product from the store

Here's how to extract Aloe vera gel directly from the plant:
Cut a mature leaf from the plant.
Wash the leaf to remove any dirt or latex.
Cut off the thorny edges and cut the leaf open.
Use a spoon to scoop out the gel.
Apply the fresh gel to your skin as needed.
Remember to perform a patch test before applying aloe vera to your face to ensure you don't have any allergic reactions. Generally, Aloe vera is safe for almost all skin

types, but individual sensitivities can vary. Stop using immediately if you feel any irritation or discomfort.

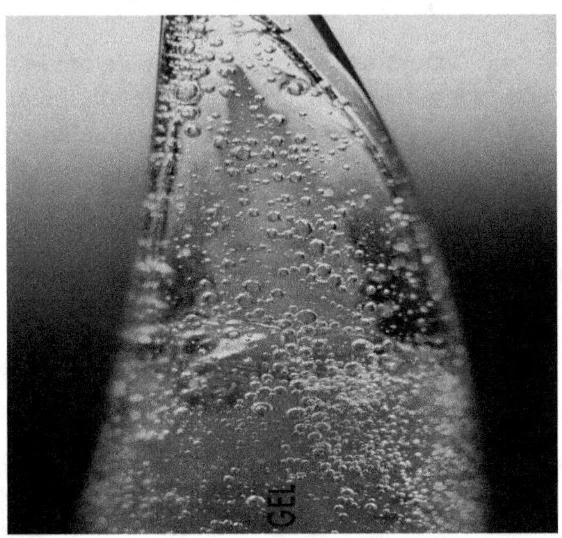

> **Clay**: Using clay for oily skin can be beneficial as its natural absorbent properties can help control excess oil, reduce shine, and unclog pores.
Some types of clay often recommended for oily skin are: Kaolin or China Clay, Bentonite Clay, French Green Clay and Rhassoul Clay

Kaolin Clay: Also known as China clay, it is a gentle and effective clay that helps absorb excess oil without overly drying the skin. All skin types, even those with sensitive skin, can use it.

Bentonite Clay: This clay has strong absorbing properties and is effective in drawing out impurities and excess oil. However, it can be quite potent, so it's

30

important not to leave it on for too long, especially if you have sensitive skin.

French Green Clay: Rich in minerals, this clay is known for its oil-absorbing and toning properties. It's particularly good for oily and combination skin.

Rhassoul Clay: Also known as Moroccan red clay, it's a versatile clay that helps absorb oil and impurities. It's less drying than some other clays, making it suitable for combination skin as well.

NOTE: When using clay for oily skin:
Frequency: Limit clay masks to once or twice a week to avoid over-drying the skin.
Application: Mix the clay with water, or aloe vera gel, or rose water to create a paste. Apply a thin layer to your face and leave it on until it's mostly dry but not completely. Rinse it off with lukewarm water.
Moisturize: Follow up with a lightweight, oil-free moisturizer to maintain the skin's hydration balance.

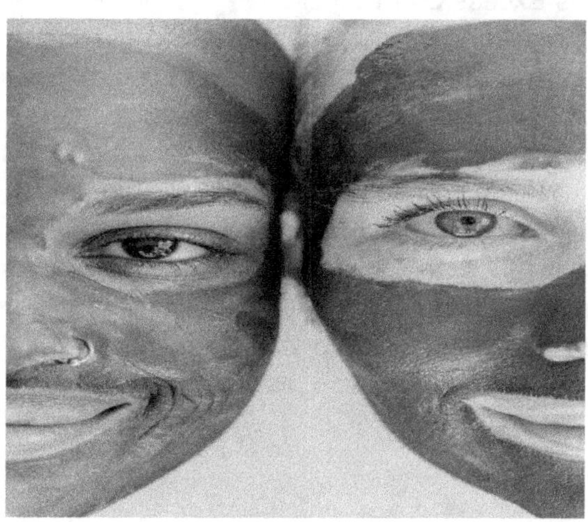

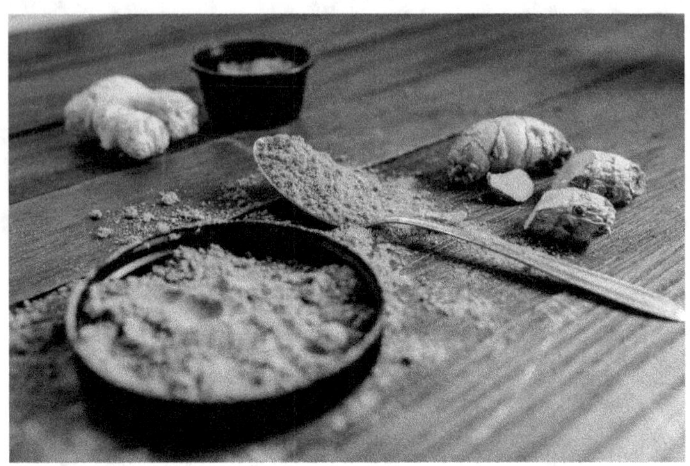

> **Turmeric:** a bright yellow spice derived from the Curcuma longa plant, has been widely recognized for its numerous health and skincare benefits. When it comes to oily skin, turmeric can be particularly advantageous due to its anti-inflammatory, antimicrobial, and antioxidant properties. Here are some of the benefits:

Controls Excess Oil Production:
Turmeric helps regulate sebum production, the oily substance produced by the skin's sebaceous glands. By controlling excess oil, turmeric can contribute to a more balanced complexion for those with oily skin.

Anti-Inflammatory Properties:
Curcumin, the active compound in turmeric, possesses powerful anti-inflammatory effects. This can be beneficial for individuals with oily skin, as inflammation is often associated with acne and other skin issues.

Antimicrobial Action:
Turmeric has natural antimicrobial and antibacterial
properties, which can be beneficial for preventing and
treating acne and other skin infections commonly
associated with oily skin.

Reduces Acne and Blemishes:
The anti-inflammatory and antibacterial properties of
turmeric make it effective in reducing acne and
blemishes. It can help soothe irritated skin and promote
a clearer complexion.

Antioxidant Protection:
Turmeric is rich in antioxidants that help protect the skin
from free radical damage. This is important for
maintaining skin health and preventing premature aging,
even for those with oily skin.

Incorporating Turmeric into Daily and Monthly Skincare
Routine:

Daily Cleansing Routine:
Add a pinch of turmeric powder to your regular face
cleanser. Mix well and use it to cleanse your face daily.
This helps in controlling oil production and promoting a
clearer complexion.

Turmeric Face Mask (1-2 times a week):
Create a DIY face mask by mixing turmeric powder with
ingredients like yogurt or honey. Apply the mask to your
face, leave it on for 15-20 minutes, and then rinse off.
This can help reduce inflammation, control oil, and
improve overall skin texture.

Turmeric and Aloe Vera Gel Spot Treatment:
Mix a small amount of turmeric with aloe vera gel and apply it as a spot treatment on acne-prone areas. This can help reduce inflammation and accelerate the healing of acne.

Turmeric and Besan (Chickpea Flour) Scrub (Once a week):
Combine turmeric with besan and a little water to create a paste. Gently scrub your face with this mixture to exfoliate the skin, removing excess oil and dead skin cells.

Turmeric-infused Moisturizer:
Mix a small amount of turmeric powder with your regular moisturizer before applying it to your face. This helps in providing the benefits of turmeric without the need for a separate step in your routine.

Turmeric and Sandalwood Powder Face Pack (Monthly):
Create a monthly face pack by combining turmeric with sandalwood powder and rose water. This can be a more intensive treatment to control oil, reduce inflammation, and promote a healthy glow.

Note: Perform a patch test before using turmeric on your face to ensure you don't have an adverse reaction. Additionally, avoid using too much turmeric, as it may temporarily stain the skin yellow.

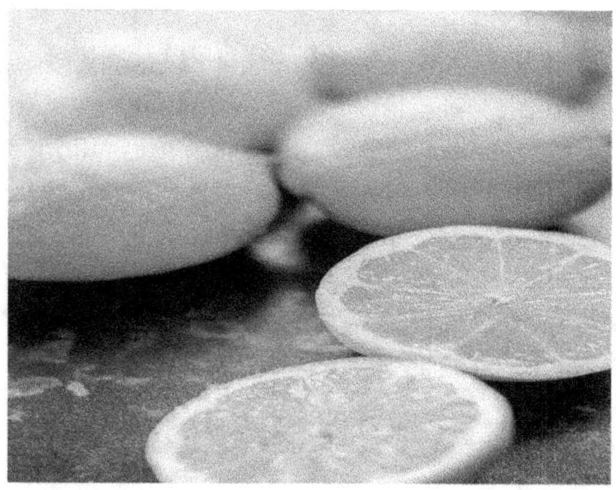

➢ **Lemon Juice**: Lemon juice contains citric acid, which can help control oil production and brighten the skin. It's advisable to dilute it with water and avoid sun exposure when using lemon juice.

Lemon juice is a popular natural ingredient that is sometimes used in skincare routines. It contains citric acid, vitamin C, and other antioxidants, which can have potential benefits for the skin. However, it's important to use lemon juice with caution and be aware of its potential drawbacks. Here are some aspects to consider:

Potential Benefits:
Vitamin C: Lemon juice is a good source of vitamin C, an antioxidant that can help brighten the skin, reduce hyperpigmentation, and promote collagen production.
Exfoliation: The citric acid in lemon juice has exfoliating properties, which can help remove dead skin cells and unclog pores, potentially reducing acne.
Lightening Properties: Some people use lemon juice to lighten dark spots or hyperpigmentation on the skin.

Caution and Considerations:
Skin Sensitivity: Lemon juice is highly acidic, and it can be harsh on the skin. If you have sensitive skin, it may cause irritation, redness, or a burning sensation. Always do a patch test before applying lemon juice to your face.

Photosensitivity: Lemon juice has the potential to increase photosensitivity, or skin sensitivity to sunlight. If you apply lemon juice to your skin, it's important to use sunscreen to protect your skin from potential sun damage.

Dryness: The acidity of lemon juice can strip the skin of natural oils, leading to dryness. If you have dry or sensitive skin, using lemon juice may exacerbate these conditions.

Dilution is Key: If you decide to use lemon juice on your skin, it's crucial to dilute it with water or mix it with other soothing ingredients like honey or aloe vera gel to reduce its acidity.

How to Use Lemon Juice in Skincare:
If you choose to incorporate lemon juice into your skincare routine, here's a simple way to use it:
Dilution: Mix lemon juice with water or other soothing ingredients. A common ratio is one part lemon juice to one part water.
Patch Test: Before applying lemon juice to your face, perform a patch test on a small area of your skin to check for any adverse reactions. Apply a small amount of the diluted mixture to a patch of skin (such as the inside of your wrist) and wait 24 hours to see if any irritation occurs.

Application: If there is no adverse reaction, you can
apply the diluted lemon juice mixture to your face using a
cotton pad. Avoid the eye area.

Sun Protection: Use sunscreen after applying lemon
juice to your skin, especially if you're going outside, as
lemon juice can increase sensitivity to sunlight.

It's critical to pay attention to your skin's needs and stop
using it if you feel any irritation.
If you have concerns about your skin or are considering
using lemon juice for specific skin issues, it's advisable
to consult with a dermatologist for personalized advice.

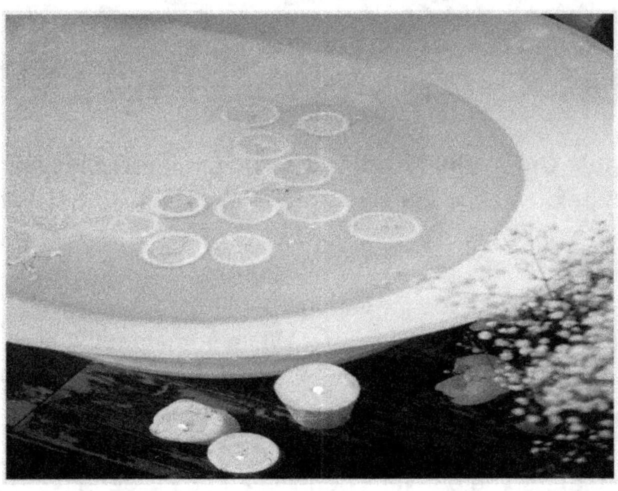

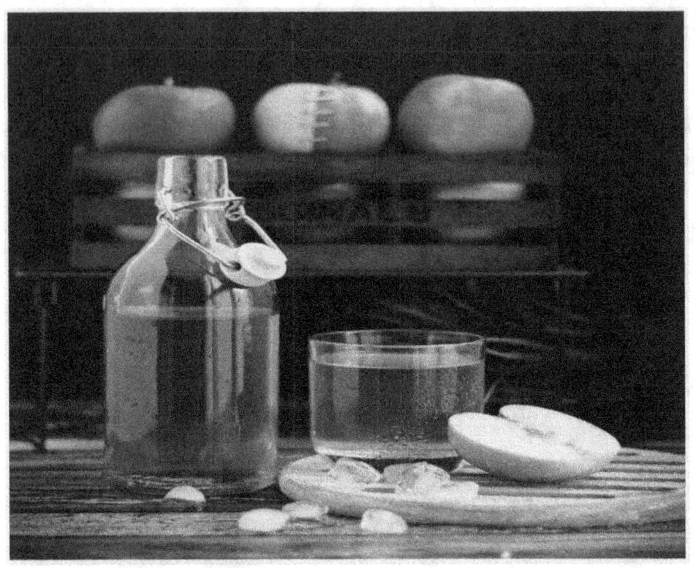

➤ **Apple Cider Vinegar**: It has astringent properties and can help balance the skin's pH levels. Dilute it with water before applying.

Apple cider vinegar (ACV) is a popular natural remedy that has been used for various health and beauty purposes, including skincare. While some people claim benefits for oily skin, it's essential to approach its use with caution, as it may not be suitable for everyone.

Here are some potential benefits and considerations when using apple cider vinegar for oily skincare:

Potential Benefits:
Balancing pH: Apple cider vinegar is slightly acidic, and it may help balance the skin's pH. Skin with an imbalanced pH may produce more oil to compensate.

Exfoliation: ACV contains acetic acid, which has exfoliating properties. This can help remove dead skin cells and unclog pores, potentially reducing excess oil.

Antibacterial Properties: ACV has some antibacterial properties, which may help control acne or breakouts associated with oily skin.

Considerations:
Dilution is Key: Apple cider vinegar is potent and can be harsh on the skin if not properly diluted. Mix it with water before applying it to your skin. A common ratio is one part ACV to three parts water.
Patch Test: Before applying it to your face, perform a patch test on a small area of your skin to ensure you don't have an adverse reaction.
Sensitivity: Some people may find ACV too harsh for their skin, leading to irritation, redness, or dryness. If you have sensitive skin, it's wise to be cautious.
Sun Sensitivity: Acidic substances can increase sensitivity to the sun. If you use ACV, it's crucial to apply sunscreen to protect your skin.

Note: Not everyone's skin reacts the same way to skincare products. Discontinue use if you experience any discomfort or skin irritation.
Consult a Professional: If you have serious skin concerns, it's always a good idea to consult with a dermatologist before trying home remedies.

How to Use:
If you decide to incorporate apple cider vinegar into your skincare routine, here's a simple way to do it:
Dilution: Mix one part apple cider vinegar with three parts water.

Application: Apply the diluted solution to your face using a cotton pad or by gently patting it onto your skin.
Frequency: Start with once a day and see how your skin reacts. You can gradually increase or decrease frequency based on your skin's response.

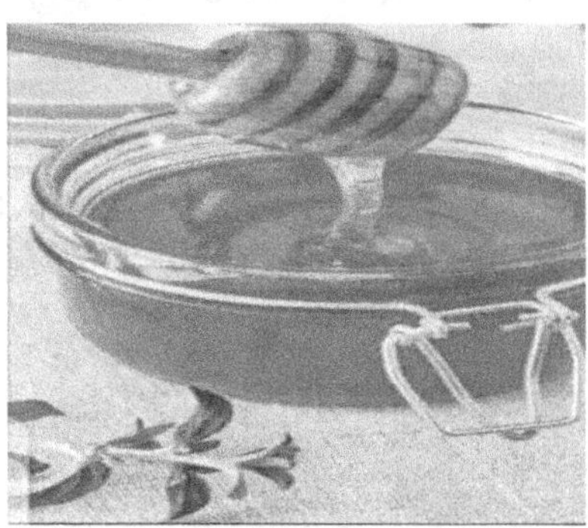

➢ **Honey:** Honey is a natural humectant, which means it can help retain moisture in the skin without making it overly oily. It also has antibacterial properties.
Honey can be a beneficial addition to your skincare routine, even if you have oily skin. It has natural antibacterial and anti-inflammatory properties, making it suitable for various skin types.

Here's how honey can be incorporated into your oily skincare routine:

Cleanser:
Mix a small amount of raw honey with water or your regular cleanser.
Gently massage it onto your face and then rinse thoroughly.
This can help cleanse the skin without stripping it of its natural oils.

Exfoliator:
Combine honey with a small amount of ground oats or
sugar to create a gentle exfoliating scrub.
Use this mixture to exfoliate your face once or twice a
week. It helps remove dead skin cells and unclog pores.

Mask:
Apply a thin layer of raw honey to your face and leave it
on for about 15-20 minutes.
Honey's antibacterial properties can help manage acne,
while its humectant properties help retain moisture.
Rinse off with warm water.
Spot Treatment:
Dab a small amount of honey onto blemishes as a spot
treatment.
The antibacterial properties can assist in reducing
inflammation and promoting healing.

Moisturizer:
In some cases, honey can be used as a light moisturizer.
Apply a small amount to your face and massage it in.
This is more suitable for those with oily skin who still
need hydration without the heaviness of some
moisturizers.

Masks with Other Ingredients:
Combine honey with ingredients like clay or yogurt for a
more targeted approach to oil control.
Clay can help absorb excess oil, while yogurt provides
additional soothing and probiotic benefits.
When using honey for skincare:
Choose Raw Honey: Raw, unprocessed honey retains
more of its beneficial properties compared to processed
honey.

Patch Test: Before applying honey to your entire face, do a patch test to ensure you don't have an allergic reaction.
Frequency: Start by incorporating honey into your routine once or twice a week to see how your skin reacts.
Quality Matters: Use high-quality honey for the best results.

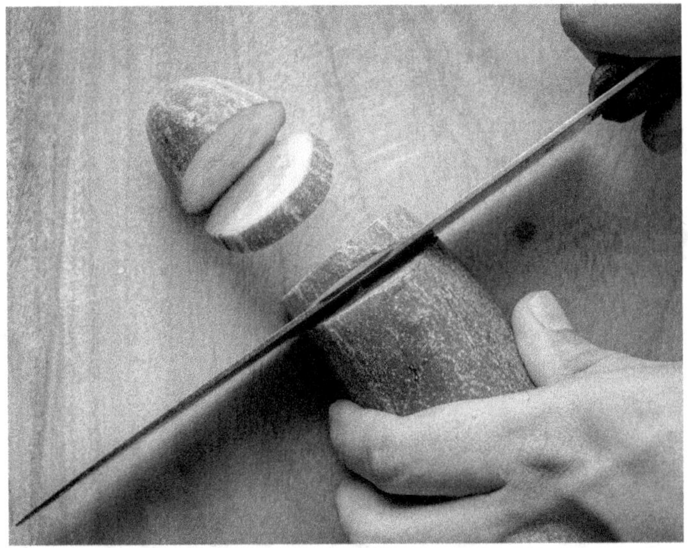

➢ **Cucumber**: Cucumber can have a cooling and soothing effect on the skin. It can also help tighten pores. Cucumbers can be beneficial for oily skin due to their natural astringent and hydrating properties.

Here are some ways in which you can use cucumbers for oily skincare:

Cucumber Slices:
Place cucumber slices on your face for about 15-20 minutes. The natural astringent properties of cucumbers can help to tighten pores and reduce excess oil

Cucumber Juice:
Extract cucumber juice and apply it to your face using a cotton ball. Allow it to sit for 15-20 minutes before rinsing with cool water. This can help control oil production.

Cucumber and Yogurt Mask:
Mix cucumber puree with plain yogurt to create a mask. Apply the mixture to your face and wait 15-20 minutes before rinsing. yogurt helps in balancing the skin's pH and has a mild exfoliating effect.
Cucumber and Lemon Mask:
Combine cucumber puree with a few drops of lemon juice. Lemon has astringent properties that can further help control oil. Apply the mask for 15-20 minutes and then rinse thoroughly.

Cucumber and Oatmeal Scrub:
Mix cucumber puree with ground oatmeal to create a gentle scrub. Exfoliating can help remove excess oil and dead skin cells. This scrub should be used once or twice a week.

Cucumber and Witch Hazel Toner:
Mix cucumber juice with witch hazel to create a natural toner. Apply the toner with a cotton pad after cleansing your face. Witch hazel is known for its astringent properties, which can help control oil.

Cucumber and Aloe Vera Gel:
Mix cucumber puree with aloe vera gel. Aloe vera has
soothing properties and can help balance the skin. Apply
the mixture and leave it on for 15-20 minutes before
rinsing.

Cucumber Ice Cubes:
Freeze cucumber juice into ice cubes and rub them on
your face in gentle, circular motions. This can reduce
oiliness and tighten pores.

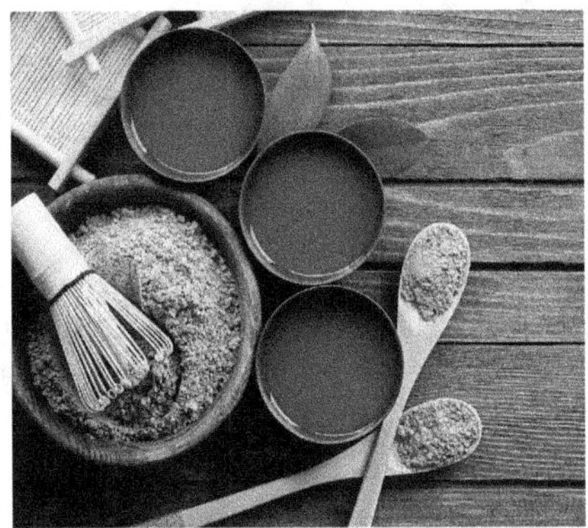

➢ **Green Tea:** Green tea contains antioxidants and can
help reduce oil production and inflammation. It can be
added to Homemade masks or used as a Toner.
Green tea can be a beneficial addition to a skincare
routine, especially for individuals with oily skin.

Here are some reasons why green tea can be helpful for
oily skin:
Antioxidant Properties: Green tea is rich in antioxidants,
such as catechins, which can help neutralize free
radicals. Free radicals can contribute to skin aging and
damage. By incorporating green tea into your skincare

routine, you may help protect your skin from oxidative stress.

Anti-Inflammatory Effects: Green tea has anti-inflammatory properties that can help soothe irritated skin. Oily skin is often associated with inflammation, and using products containing green tea may help calm the skin and reduce redness.

Regulation of Sebum Production: Some studies suggest that green tea may help regulate sebum (oil) production in the skin. Excessive sebum production can contribute to oily skin and may lead to issues such as acne. Green tea may help balance oil production without over-drying the skin.

Acne-Fighting Properties: The anti-inflammatory and antibacterial properties of green tea may also be beneficial for those dealing with acne. It can help prevent and treat acne lesions, making it a good option for those with oily, acne-prone skin.

Here's how you can incorporate green tea into your skincare routine for oily skin:

Green Tea Cleanser: Use a gentle cleanser containing green tea extract to clean your face. This can help remove excess oil and impurities while providing antioxidant benefits.

Green Tea Toner: Apply a green tea-infused toner to balance your skin's pH levels and provide additional antioxidants.

Green Tea Moisturizer: Use a lightweight, non-comedogenic moisturizer with green tea extract to hydrate your skin without clogging pores.

Green Tea Masks: Consider using a green tea mask once or twice a week to provide a concentrated dose of antioxidants and soothe the skin.
Sunscreen with Green Tea: Use a broad-spectrum sunscreen with added green tea extract to protect your skin from UV damage while benefiting from the antioxidant properties of green tea.

➤ **Oatmeal**: Oatmeal can be used as an exfoliant and can help absorb excess oil while soothing the skin.
Oatmeal can be beneficial for oily skin due to its various properties, such as being absorbent and soothing.

Here are some ways you can incorporate oatmeal into your skincare routine for oily skin:

Oatmeal Mask:
Mix finely ground oatmeal with water or aloe vera gel to create a paste.
Apply paste to your face and leave it on for 15 to 20 minutes
Rinse it off with lukewarm water.

Oatmeal and Honey Mask:
Combine finely ground oatmeal with honey to create a mask.
Smear mixture on your face and let it sit for about 15 minutes.
Rinse it off with lukewarm water.

Oatmeal Cleanser:
Mix ground oatmeal with a gentle cleanser or water to
create a paste.
Apply the paste to your face and gently massage it in
circular motions.
Rinse thoroughly with water.

Oatmeal and Yogurt Mask:
Mix ground oatmeal with plain yogurt to form a mask.
Apply paste to your face and leave it on for 15 to 20
minutes
Rinse off with lukewarm water.

Oatmeal Scrub:
Combine ground oatmeal with a bit of water to make a
scrub.
Gently massage the scrub onto your face, focusing on
areas with excess oil.
Rinse off with lukewarm water.

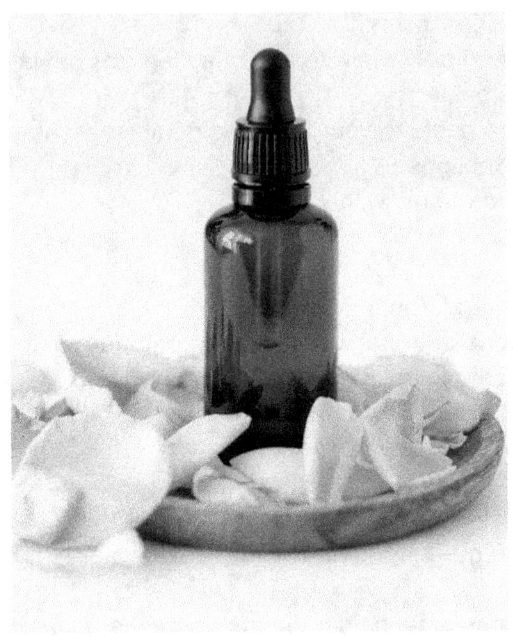

➤ **Rosewater:** Rosewater is a gentle toner that can help maintain the skin's pH balance.
Rosewater can be a beneficial addition to a skincare routine, including for individuals with oily skin.

Here are some potential benefits and ways you can incorporate rosewater into your oily skincare routine:
Hydration: Rosewater is known for its hydrating properties. Even oily skin needs hydration, as dehydration can lead to overproduction of oil. Applying rosewater can help maintain the skin's moisture balance.

Balancing pH: Rosewater has a slightly acidic pH, which can help balance the natural pH of the skin. Balanced skin is less prone to excessive oil production.

Anti-inflammatory: Rosewater has anti-inflammatory properties, which can be helpful for calming irritated skin. This is particularly beneficial for those with oily skin, as excessive oil production can sometimes be associated with inflammation.

Toning: Rosewater can act as a natural toner, helping to tighten pores. This can be beneficial for individuals with oily skin, as enlarged pores can contribute to excess oil production.

Here's how you can incorporate rosewater into your oily skincare routine:

Cleansing: Use rosewater as a gentle cleanser. You can mix it with a small amount of your regular cleanser or use it on its own to remove impurities.

Toning: Apply rosewater as a toner after cleansing. You can either spray it directly onto your face or use a cotton pad to apply it.

Moisturizing: Follow up with a lightweight, oil-free moisturizer to lock in the hydration from the rosewater.

Makeup Setting Spray: Rosewater can also be used as a natural makeup setting spray. This can help control excess shine throughout the day.

It's essential to choose a high-quality, pure rosewater without added preservatives or synthetic fragrances. Additionally, while rosewater can be beneficial, it's not a standalone solution. It should be part of a comprehensive skincare routine that includes cleansing, moisturizing, and sun protection.

CAUTION:

When using these natural ingredients, it's essential to perform a patch test first to ensure you don't have any adverse reactions. Additionally, if you have a severe skin condition, it's a good idea to consult with a dermatologist before making any significant changes to your skincare routine.

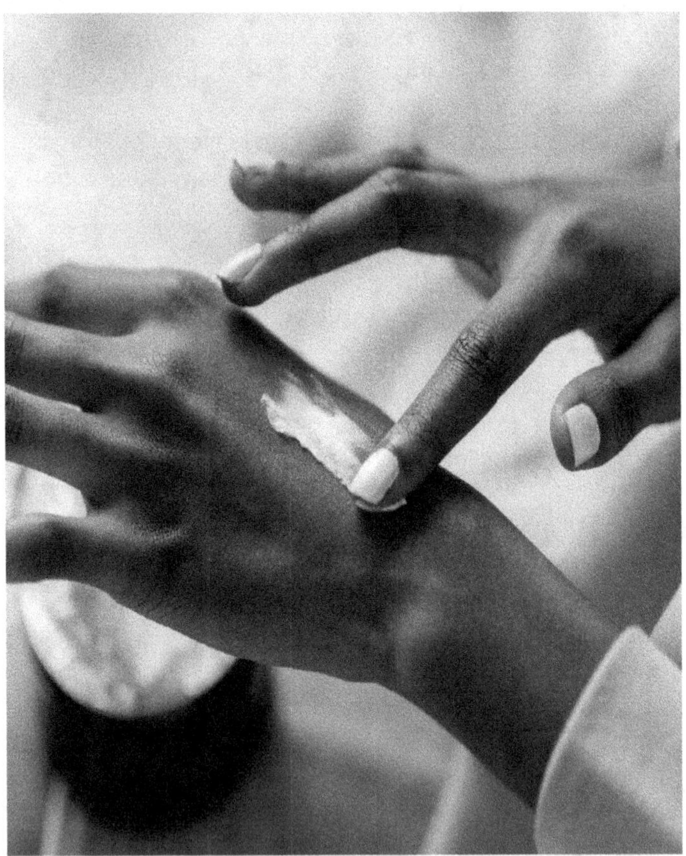

CHAPTER SIX

LIFESTYLE TIPS FOR MANAGING OILY SKIN

Managing oily skin requires a combination of proper skincare, lifestyle choices, and possibly adjustments to your daily routine. Here are some tips to help you manage oily skin:
Cleanse regularly:

Wash your face twice a day, in the morning and before bed, with a mild, oil-free cleanser.
Avoid harsh or abrasive cleansers, as they can strip your skin of essential oils, leading to increased oil production.

Use oil-free products:
Choose oil-free or non-comedogenic (won't clog pores) moisturizers, sunscreens, and makeup products.
Look for products with labels like "oil-free," "non-comedogenic," or "water-based."

Hydrate:
Don't skip moisturizing, even if you have oily skin. Opt for oil-free or gel-based moisturizers to keep your skin hydrated without adding excess oil.

Exfoliate regularly:
Exfoliate your skin 1-2 times a week to remove dead skin cells and prevent clogged pores. Look for products with salicylic acid or glycolic acid.

Use a clay mask:
Clay masks can help absorb excess oil and reduce shine. Use them once or twice a week to keep your skin balanced.

Avoid touching your face:
Touching your face can transfer oil, dirt, and bacteria, leading to breakouts. Try to avoid touching your face throughout the day.

Choose the right makeup:
Use oil-free and non-comedogenic makeup products. Mineral makeup can be a good option as it tends to be lighter and less likely to clog pores.

Stay hydrated:
Drink plenty of water to help flush out toxins and keep your skin hydrated from the inside.

Balanced diet:
Consume a diet rich in fruits, vegetables, and whole grains. Avoid excessive consumption of greasy or fried foods, as they can contribute to oily skin.

Manage stress:
Stress can trigger an increase in oil production. Practice stress-reducing activities such as yoga, meditation, or deep breathing exercises.

Regular exercise:
Regular physical activity helps regulate hormones and can contribute to healthier skin. Remember to cleanse your face after exercising to remove sweat and oil
Get enough sleep:

Lack of sleep can contribute to increased stress and hormone levels, which may lead to oilier skin. Aim for 7-9 hours of quality sleep each night.
If you find that these tips do not effectively manage your oily skin, or if your skin condition worsens, it's advisable to consult with a dermatologist for personalized advice and potential medical treatments.

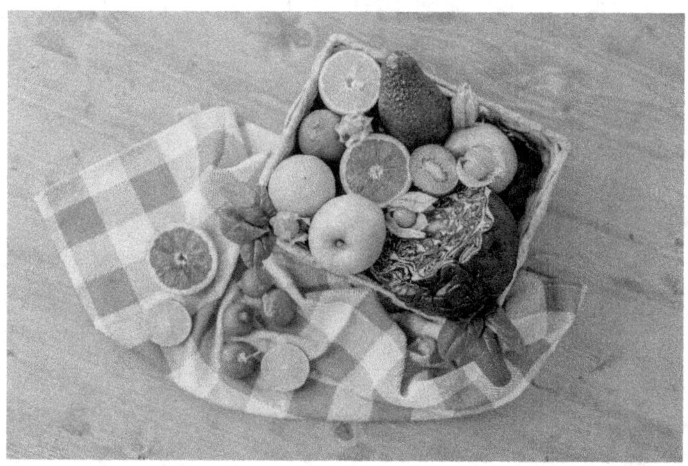

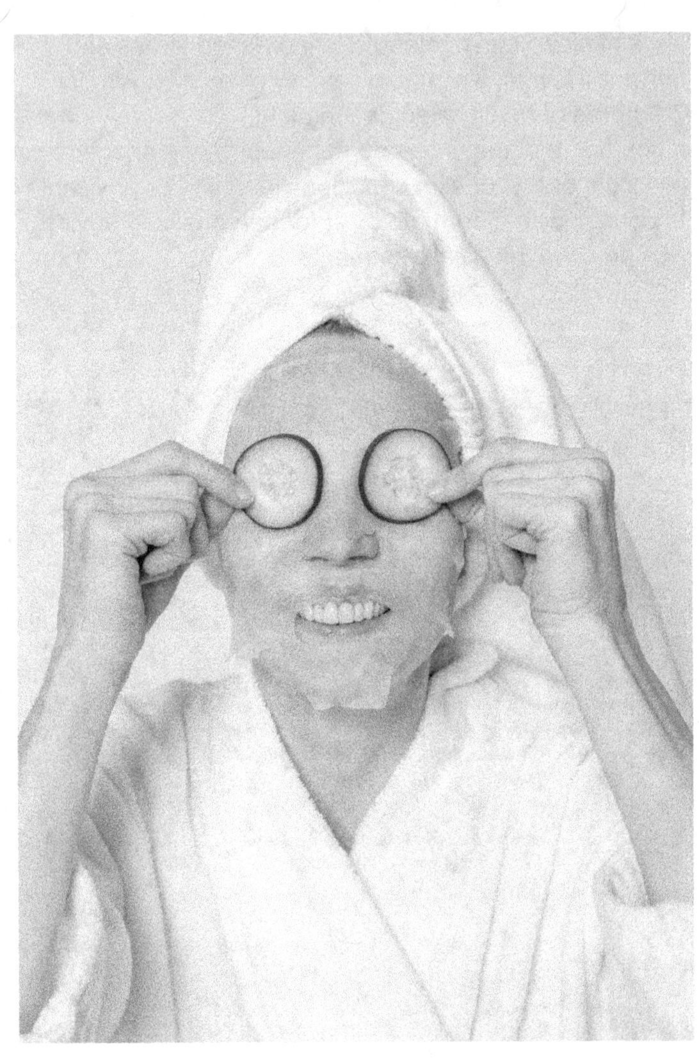

CHAPTER SEVEN

COMMON MISTAKES

Managing oily skin can be challenging, and it's important to avoid certain common mistakes to maintain a healthy complexion. Here are some mistakes to avoid in oily skincare management:

Overwashing the Face: Washing your face too frequently or using harsh cleansers.
Why it's bad: Overwashing can strip the skin of its natural oils, leading to increased oil production as the skin tries to compensate.

Skipping Moisturizer:
 Avoiding moisturizer because of concerns about adding more oil to the skin.
Why it's bad: All skin types, including oily skin, need hydration. Skipping moisturizer can lead to dehydrated skin, causing the oil glands to produce more oil to compensate.

Using Harsh Products:
 Using overly harsh or abrasive skincare products.
Why it's bad: Harsh products can irritate the skin and trigger increased oil production. Opt for gentle, non-comedogenic products that won't clog pores.

Sunscreen:
 Neglecting sunscreen in your skincare routine.
Why it's bad: Sun damage can worsen oily skin and contribute to premature aging. Choose a

non-comedogenic, broad-spectrum sunscreen to protect
your skin.

Picking at the Skin:
Picking, squeezing, or popping pimples.
Why it's bad: This can lead to inflammation, scarring,
and the spread of bacteria. It may also stimulate more oil
production.

Using Heavy, Oil-Based Products:
 Using thick, oil-based products.
Why it's bad: Heavy products can clog pores and
contribute to breakouts. Look for oil-free,
non-comedogenic options.

Not Exfoliating Regularly:
 Neglecting regular exfoliation.
Why it's bad: Exfoliation helps remove dead skin cells
and unclog pores, preventing the buildup of excess oil.
Use a gentle exfoliant, such as salicylic acid, a few times
a week.

Consistent Routine:
Mistake: Inconsistency in your skincare routine.
Why it's bad: Consistency is key for skincare. Regular
cleansing, moisturizing, and sun protection help manage
oil production and maintain a balanced complexion.

Using Alcohol-Based Products:
 Using products with high concentrations of alcohol.
Why it's bad: Alcohol can be excessively drying and may
irritate the skin, leading to increased oil production as
the skin tries to compensate.

Neglecting Professional Advice:
Not seeking advice from a dermatologist.
Why it's bad: If you're struggling with persistent oily skin issues, it's advisable to consult a dermatologist. They can provide personalized recommendations and address underlying issues.

Remember that everyone's skin is unique, so it may take some trial and error to find the best routine for your oily skin. If you're uncertain about the products or methods that will work best for you, consulting with a skincare professional is always a good idea

INGREDIENTS TO AVOID FOR OILY SKIN

If you have oily skin, it's important to be mindful of the ingredients in your skincare and makeup products to avoid exacerbating the issue. Here are some common ingredients to avoid or use with caution if you have oily skin:

Alcohol: Avoid products with high concentrations of alcohol, as they can strip your skin of natural oils, leading to increased oil production to compensate.

Fragrance: Fragrances can sometimes irritate the skin, which may lead to increased oil production. Look for fragrance-free or hypoallergenic products.

Mineral Oil and Petrolatum: These ingredients can be heavy and clog pores, potentially causing breakouts in individuals with oily skin.

Silicones: While not necessarily harmful, some people find that silicone-based products can feel heavy on the skin and trap oil underneath, leading to a greasy appearance.

Comedogenic Ingredients: Look for non-comedogenic products. These are less prone to clogging pores and causing breakouts. While many natural ingredients are beneficial for oily skin, some may exacerbate the issue. It's advisable to steer clear of heavy oils like coconut oil, Shea Butter and Cocoa Butter which can clog pores, and overly rich moisturizers that may contribute to an unwanted sheen

Sulfates: Sulfates, like sodium lauryl sulfate, are commonly found in cleansers and can be harsh on the skin. They can strip away natural oils, potentially causing an increase in oil production.
Heavy, Creamy Moisturizers: While moisturizing is essential for all skin types, very thick or greasy moisturizer can make oily skin feel even oilier. Opt for lightweight, oil-free, or gel-based moisturizers.

Overly Harsh Exfoliants: While exfoliating is important for oily skin to prevent clogged pores, avoid using products with very abrasive or sharp particles that can damage the skin. Chemical exfoliants with salicylic acid or glycolic acid are often better choices.

Occlusive Products: Products that create a heavy barrier on the skin, like some night creams and ointments, can trap oil and heat, making oily skin worse. Opt for lighter, oil-free options.

Hydrating Ingredients: Oily skin still needs hydration, but opt for products with ingredients like hyaluronic acid or glycerin, which provide hydration without adding excess oil.

Waxes: Waxy ingredients like beeswax can be heavy and may contribute to a greasy feeling on the skin. It's important to note that individual skin types and sensitivities can vary, so what works for one person with oily skin may not work for another. If you're uncertain about specific products, consider doing a patch test or consulting with a dermatologist or skincare professional to find the best products for your skin type. Additionally, maintaining a consistent and gentle skincare routine is crucial for managing oily skin.

DEALING WITH OILY SKIN CONCERNS

Managing acne and blemishes for oily skin requires a consistent and targeted skincare routine. Oily skin is prone to excess sebum production, which can give rise to some skin concerns such as Acne, Excess shine, Enlarged pores and Blemishes.
Managing these concerns in oily skin involves a combination of proper, consistent and targeted skincare routine, lifestyle changes, and, in some cases, professional treatments. Note that individual responses to treatments may vary, and it's always a good idea to consult with a dermatologist for personalized advice. Here's a comprehensive guide to help you manage these concerns:

1. Cleanse Regularly:
Use a gentle, oil-free cleanser with salicylic acid or
benzoyl peroxide to help control acne.
Cleanse your face twice a day, in the morning and
before bedtime, to remove excess oil and impurities.

2. Exfoliate:
Incorporate exfoliation into your routine to prevent
clogged pores and remove dead skin cells.
Use a salicylic acid or glycolic acid exfoliant 2-3 times a
week.

3. Moisturize:
Even oily skin needs hydration. Choose a
non-comedogenic, oil-free moisturizer to keep the skin
balanced.
Hydrating the skin can actually help regulate oil
production.

4. Sun Protection:
Use a broad-spectrum sunscreen with at least SPF 30
daily to protect your skin from UV damage.
Look for oil-free or gel-based sunscreens to avoid
adding excess oil to your skin.

5. Topical Treatments:
Consider using over-the-counter products with
ingredients like benzoyl peroxide, salicylic acid, or
retinoids to control acne.
Apply spot treatments directly on acne-prone areas.

6. Healthy Diet:
Consume a healthy diet that is high in fruits, vegetables,
and whole grains.

Limit intake of high-glycemic foods and dairy, as they
may contribute to acne.

7. Stay Hydrated:
For the sake of your general health and skin hydration,
drink lots of water.

8. Avoid Touching Your Face:
Acne can worsen when you touch your face because it
transfers oil and bacteria from your hands to your skin.

9. Use Oil-Absorbing Products:
Select makeup and skincare products that are labeled
"oil-free" or "non-comedogenic."
Consider using oil-absorbing sheets throughout the day
to control shine.

10. Professional Treatments:
Consult with a dermatologist for professional treatments
like chemical peels, microdermabrasion, or laser therapy
to address acne and pore size.

11. Lifestyle Changes:
Manage stress through practices like yoga or meditation,
as stress can contribute to acne.
Ensure you get adequate sleep for overall skin health.

12. Avoid Harsh Scrubs:
Harsh physical scrubs can irritate the skin and worsen
acne. Stick to gentle exfoliants.

13. Patience is Key:
Skincare routines take time to show results. Be patient
and consistent with your routine.

Remember, everyone's skin is unique, and it may take some trial and error to find the right combination of products and routines that work for you. If your acne is persistent or severe, seeking professional advice is crucial.

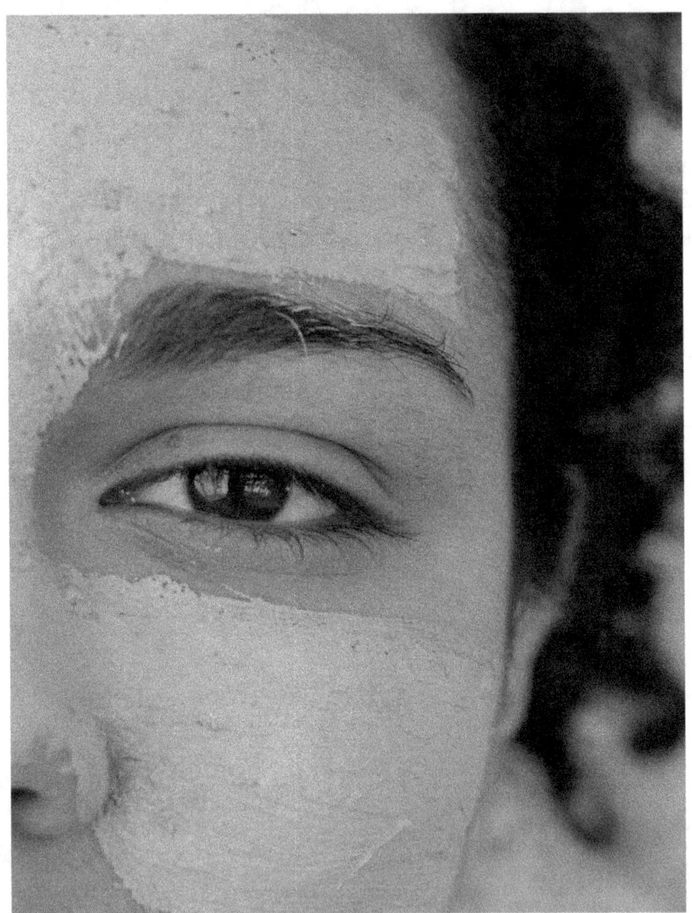

Conclusion:

In your journey to achieving balanced and radiant skin, embracing natural ingredients tailored to oily skin is a wise choice. Consistency is key, so incorporate these ingredients into your daily and weekly routine, and soon you'll find your skin thanking you for the gentle, natural care it deserves. Remember, achieving healthy skin is a journey, and with nature as your ally, you're well on your way to a naturally beautiful complexion.

Remember that everyone's skin is different, so what works for one person may not work the same way for another. It's critical to pay attention to your skin's needs and modify your skincare regimen as necessary. If you experience any irritation or discomfort while using any homemade recipe or skincare product, discontinue use and consult a healthcare professional. However, do not forget to always do a patch test first before use.

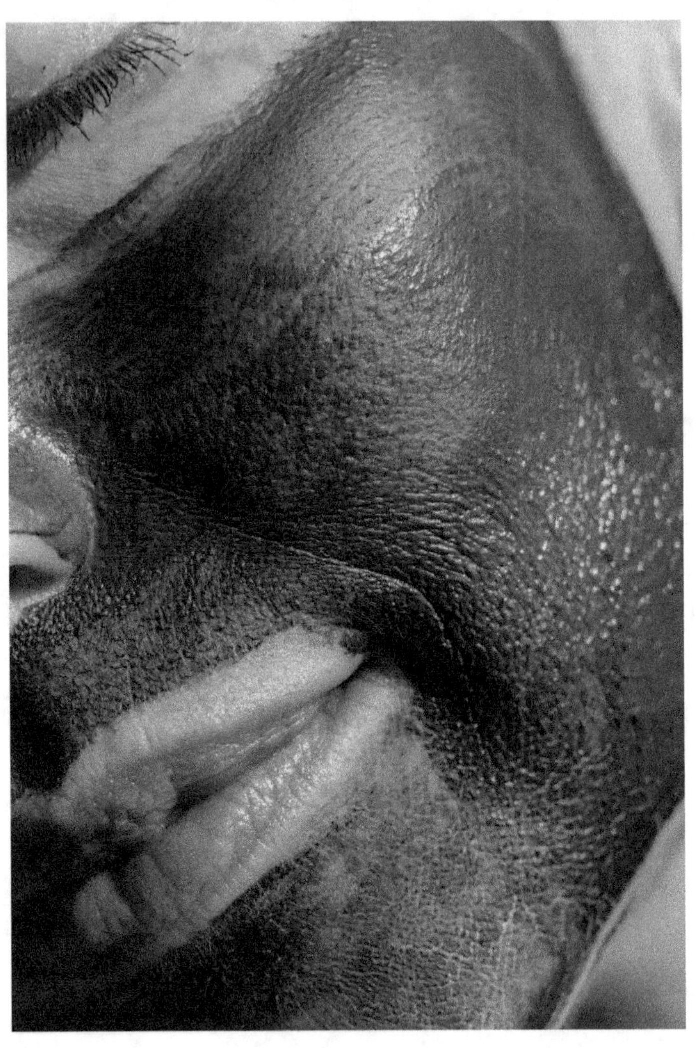